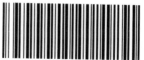

EMT
Pocket Review

EMT
Pocket Review

Stephen Marc Szabo, EMT
Firefighter, Merrimac Fire Department
Merrimac, Massachusetts

Foreword by Captain William Haug, EMT, EMT IC
Portsmouth Naval Shipyard Fire Department
Portsmouth, New Hampshire
Director, Prehospital Care Program
Northern Essex Community College
Haverhill, Massachusetts

Little, Brown and Company
Boston   New York   Toronto   London

Library of Congress Cataloging-in-Publication Data

Szabo, Stephen Marc.
    EMT pocket review / Stephen Marc Szabo.
        p.   cm.
    ISBN 0-316-82415-1
    1. Emergency medicine—Handbooks, manuals, etc. 2. Emergency
medicine—Outlines, syllabi, etc. 3. Emergency medical technicians.
I. Title.
    [DNLM: 1. Emergency Medical Services—handbooks. 2. Emergency
Medical Technicians—education—handbooks. WX 39 S996e 1995]
RC86.8.S96   1995
616.02'5'076—dc20
DNLM/DLC
for Library of Congress   94-44576
                                                               CIP

Printed in the United States of America
RRD-VA

Editorial: Evan R. Schnittman, Suzanne Jeans
Production Editor: Marie A. Salter
Production Supervisor/Designer: Michael A. Granger
Cover Designer: Michael A. Granger

Contents

Foreword

An individual who becomes an emergency medical technician (EMT) has elected one of the toughest professions in the world. An EMT is duty-bound and morally obligated to provide the best prehospital care he or she can to the patient. Split-second decisions affecting the patient's well-being must be made, often under adverse conditions. Once the EMT has arrived on the scene and begun to render aid, there is no time to "look it up" in a book. The principles of emergency care must be so completely understood and thoroughly ingrained that the EMT does not have to think, just react. The EMT must be master of patient assessment and other skills so that the patient, properly managed, stabilized, and transported, can receive definitive care.

The purpose of this book is twofold. First, it will help the EMT student prepare for the written and practical certification examinations in his or her state. Second, the book will serve as a lifelong study guide and reference and will aid in the retention of skills that may not be used on a regular basis.

Anyone who accepts the challenge of becoming an EMT will find gratification if he or she is mentally prepared to provide the best possible prehospital medical care for the patient.

Captain William Haug

Preface

It is gratifying for me to see this study aid being published. While taking the course to become an EMT, I had considerable difficulty finding the time and means to study and memorize the vital information necessary to pass the state exam and, more important, to be able to identify and properly treat patients when on the street. I was also concerned about how long I would retain the information I learned, even with all of the continuing education opportunities available. When I decided to put together these "bites" of information for my own use, I thought they might help. By the time I finished, however, I realized they would be the key to my passing the state exam and building my confidence in the future. I hope *EMT Pocket Review* will do the same for you.

The book is divided into two parts, which correspond to the two parts of the certification exam. In the first part, The Written Exam, conditions are grouped by type and body region. Signs and symptoms and management are given for each condition, and helpful mnemonics supplement the text. The second part, The Practical Exam, presents the stations you will encounter in the practical and highlights the steps you must do correctly in order to pass each specific station. Although *EMT Pocket Review* contains all the information you need to pass the written and practical state certification exams, it is intended first and foremost as a study aid and review book and should be used in conjunction with major texts in the field.

I am happy to have the opportunity to pass this book along to you and am confident you will use it throughout your years of service as an EMT, be it on a volunteer, on-call, or full-time service basis.

S.M.S.

Acknowledgments

First, I extend my appreciation to Jim Roy, for the countless hours he spent applying his literary talents to this project.

I also thank Bill Haug, for the instruction and guidance that led to my writing this book, and also for the many hours he spent exercising his expertise and memory when reviewing the manuscript.

To the Merrimac Fire Department and all its members, I extend a special thanks for all they have done to promote me as an active member in the firefighting and emergency medical services fields.

I am grateful to the many people who have shared their knowledge and resources with me through the various continuing education courses I have attended, in particular to the instructors at Water Education Training for their contribution.

To the people at Little, Brown and Company — my editor, Evan Schnittman, editorial assistant, Suzanne Jeans, and production editor, Marie Salter — and to reviewer Jeffrey Barrow, my appreciation for all their hard work.

To my good friend Keith Frosnock, thanks for his support and help during this project.

For their interest and encouragement, my parents deserve special mention.

And most of all, I thank my wife, Alison, and daughter, Emily, for their patience, understanding, and support during the long hours I spent working on this project. I look forward to spending those hours with them now.

I

The Written Exam

The written portion of the EMT certification exam is multiple choice. The time allotted and number of questions in the written exam vary from state to state, but most of the vital information you need to know is covered in this section.

The questions asked in the written exam deal with hypothetical signs and symptoms—you must determine the most appropriate treatment. For example, a question may read:

A middle-aged man is hit by a car, which throws him about ten feet away. When you arrive at the scene, the man is unconscious and lying in a pool of blood. There is definite deformity of the left femur, and the left trouser leg is soaked in blood. In what order should the following steps be taken?

a. Transport the patient.	1. _____
b. Determine that there is a pulse.	2. _____
c. Complete the secondary survey.	3. _____
d. Expose the injured leg.	4. _____
e. Apply traction splint to the injured leg.	5. _____
f. Determine that the patient is breathing.	6. _____
g. Apply direct pressure to the wound on leg.	7. _____
h. Administer oxygen.	8. _____
i. Immobilize patient on long board.	9. _____
j. Open and clear airway.	10. _____
k. Hold injured leg in manual traction.	11. _____

The correct answer is *j, f, b, d, g, h, k, e, i, c, a.*

Another type of question you might see is oriented toward less obvious medical symptoms. For example,

You get a call that a man is staggering down the street. When you arrive, you find a forty-year-old man who is disoriented and combative; his speech is slurred, and he is drooling. His skin is cold and clammy. His BP is 110/60, and his respirations are 16 and unlabored. What would you suspect his problem to be?

a. Pneumonia
b. Hypoglycemia
c. Hernia
d. Traumatic asphyxia

The correct answer is *b.*

As you can see, the questions in the written exam vary in difficulty as well as content. The information in this section will help you prepare for any questions you may be asked.

1
Shock

General Signs

Signs and Symptoms	Management
Diminished LOC (*level of c*onsciousness)	ABE M HOT RN
Confusion, anxiety, restlessness	1. Airway, open and clear.
Fear of dying	2. Bleeding, control.
Pale, cold and clammy skin	3. Elevate feet 12–18 in.
Diaphoresis (heavy sweating)	4. Maintain temperature.
Nausea and vomiting	5. Handle with care.
Intense thirst	6. O_2, administer.
Shallow, rapid respirations	7. Transport.
Dilated pupils	8. Reassure.
Weak and rapid pulse	9. Nothing by mouth.
Diminished capillary refill	10. Take vitals every 5 minutes. 🕐
Blood pressure drops	

Anaphylactic Shock

Signs and Symptoms	Management
HICCEL	1. Open and clear airway.
Hives	2. Administer O_2.
Itching	3. Rapid transport!
Cyanosis (blue skin)	
Constriction of chest	4. Take vitals every 5 minutes. 🕐
Edema of lips and tongue	
Laryngeal spasm	

Cardiogenic Shock

Signs and Symptoms	Management

Signs and Symptoms

Chest pain, nonspecific and/or dull

Dyspnea (shortness of breath)

Weak and rapid pulse

Cyanosis (blue skin)

Diminished LOC (*level of c*onsciousness)

Lowered distal pulse

Cold and clammy skin

Denial

Fear of dying

Management

ABE M HOT RN

1. **A**irway, open and clear.
2. **B**leeding, control.
3. **E**levate feet 12–18 in.
4. **M**aintain temperature.
5. **H**andle with care.
6. **O**$_2$, administer.
7. **T**ransport.
8. **R**eassure.
9. **N**othing by mouth.
10. Take vitals every 5 minutes. 🕐

Hemorrhagic Shock

Signs and Symptoms	Management
Diminished LOC (*level of c*onsciousness)	**ABE M HOT RN**
Confusion, anxiety, restlessness	1. **A**irway, open and clear.
Fear of dying	2. **B**leeding, control.
Cold and clammy skin	3. **E**levate feet 12–18 in.
Diaphoresis (heavy sweating)	4. **M**aintain temperature.
Nausea and vomiting	5. **H**andle with care.
Intense thirst	6. **O**$_2$, administer.
Pale	7. **T**ransport.
Shallow, rapid respirations	8. **R**eassure.
Possible fainting	9. **N**othing by mouth.
Dilated pupils	
Weak and rapid pulse	10. Take vitals every 5 minutes.
Diminished capillary refill	
Blood pressure drops	

Psychogenic Shock

Signs and Symptoms	Management
Patient faints	1. Self-correcting; lay patient down.
Sudden drop in blood pressure	

Septic Shock

Signs and Symptoms	Management

Signs and Symptoms

History of bacterial
  infection
Elevated body
  temperature
Diminished LOC (*level
  of* consciousness)
Confusion, anxiety,
  restlessness
Fear of dying
Cold and clammy skin
Diaphoresis (heavy
  sweating)
Nausea and vomiting
Intense thirst
Pale
Shallow, rapid
  respirations
Possible syncope
  (fainting)
Dilated pupils
Weak and rapid pulse
Diminished capillary
  refill
Blood pressure drops

Management

ABE M HOT RN
1. **A**irway, open and clear.
2. **B**leeding, control.
3. **E**levate feet 12–18 in.
4. **M**aintain temperature.
5. **H**andle with care.
6. **O**$_2$, administer.
7. **T**ransport.
8. **R**eassure.
9. **N**othing by mouth.

10. Take vitals
    every 5 minutes. ⏱

2
Head

Cerebral Contusion

Signs and Symptoms	Management
Extended loss of consciousness	1. Open and clear airway: modified jaw thrust.
Limited loss of memory	2. C-spine precautions.
Varied range of paralysis, unilateral to total	3. Control bleeding, if any.*
	4. Administer high-flow O_2.
Pupils vary in dilation	5. Assist breathing, as necessary.
Deterioration of vital signs	6. Transport.
Nausea and vomiting	7. Take vitals every 5 minutes. 🕐

*Do not stop blood or cerebral spinal fluid (CSF) flow from ears or nose.

Cerebral Vascular Accident (CVA or Stroke)

Signs and Symptoms	Management
Broken or slurred speech	1. Open and clear airway.
Hemiparesis (half the body is weak)	2. Administer high-flow O_2.
	3. Take vitals.
Hemiplegia (half the body is paralyzed)	4. Rapid transport! Elevate head, if conscious; if unconscious, transport lateral recumbent, affected side down.
Uncoordinated motor function	
High BP, slowing pulse	5. Maintain temperature.
Diminished sight on one side	6. Protect affected side.
Nausea and vomiting	7. Take vitals every 5 minutes. 🕐
Stiff neck	
Sudden loss of consciousness	
Polydipsia (drooling)	

Concussion

Signs and Symptoms	Management
Short-term loss of memory concerning injury	1. Open and clear airway.
Loss of balance	2. C-spine precautions.
Possible loss of consciousness	3. Control bleeding, if any.
Seizures	4. Administer high-flow O_2.
Confusion	5. Take vitals.
	6. Assist breathing, as necessary.
	7. Rapid transport!
	8. Take vitals every 5 minutes. ⏰

Epileptic Seizure (Grand Mal)

Signs and Symptoms	Management
Loss of consciousness	1. Prevent patient from self-injury.
Periods of uncontrollable convulsions; each convulsion may last up to 60 seconds.	2. Do not restrain.
	3. Bite stick; check local protocol.
Possible incontinence	4. Open and clear airway, if possible. Do not force mouth open!
Possible cyanosis (blue skin)	5. Position lateral recumbent, if possible.
Total elapsed time of episode is generally 5 minutes.	6. Administer O_2.
	7. Take history.
	8. Take vitals.
	9. Check for injury.
	10. Maintain temperature.
	11. Transport.
	12. Take vitals every 5 minutes. ⏰

Fractured Skull

Signs and Symptoms	Management
Lumps, bumps, or indentations Blood or fluid from ears or nose Raccoon eyes (black eyes) Battle's sign (black and blue behind ears) Pupils vary in dilation	1. Open and clear airway: modified jaw thrust. 2. C-spine precautions. 3. Control soft tissue bleeding, if any.* 4. Administer high-flow O$_2$. 5. Assist breathing, as necessary. 6. Rapid transport! 7. Take vitals every 5 minutes. 🕐

*Do not stop blood or cerebral spinal fluid (CSF) flow from ears or nose. No pressure to exposed brain tissue.

Hematoma, Epidural

Signs and Symptoms	Management
Patient loses then regains consciousness, followed by diminished LOC (*level of consciousness*) Seizures Pupil on injured side fixed and dilated	1. Open and clear airway: modified jaw thrust. 2. C-spine precautions. 3. Take vitals. 4. Administer high-flow O$_2$. 5. Assist breathing, as necessary. 6. Rapid transport! 7. Take vitals every 5 minutes. 🕐

Hematoma, Subdural

Signs and Symptoms	Management
Diminished LOC (*level of c*onsciousness)	1. Open and clear airway: modified jaw thrust.
Pupils vary in dilation	2. C-spine precautions.
Nausea and vomiting	3. Take vitals.
Reversed vitals (hypertension with slowing pulse)	4. Administer high-flow O_2.
	5. Assist breathing, as necessary.
Abnormal respirations	6. Rapid transport!
	7. Take vitals every 5 minutes. 🕐

Status Epilepticus

Signs and Symptoms	Management
Loss of consciousness	1. Prevent patient from self-injury.
Periods of uncontrollable convulsions; each convulsion may last up to 60 seconds.	2. Do not restrain.
	3. Bite stick; check local protocol.
No postical (recovery) period between episodes	4. Open and clear airway, if possible.
	5. Position lateral recumbent, if possible.
Possible cyanosis (blue skin)	6. Rapid transport!
Possible incontinence	7. Administer high-flow O_2, if possible.
	8. Take vitals every 5 minutes. 🕐

Transient Ischemic Attack (TIA)

Signs and Symptoms

Broken or slurred speech
  pattern
Uncoordinated motor
  function
Hemiparesis (half the
  body is weak)
Hemiplegia (half the
  body is paralyzed)
Diminished sight in one
  eye
Syncope (fainting)
Symptoms intermittent;
  1–24 hours' duration;
  increasing in severity
  over period of days

Management

1. Open and clear airway.
2. Administer high-flow O_2.
3. Take vitals.
4. Rapid transport! Elevated head
   or semireclined position.
5. Maintain temperature.
6. Protect affected side.

7. Take vitals
   every 5 minutes. 🕐

3
Neck and Chest

General Chest Injury

Signs and Symptoms	Management
Dyspnea (shortness of breath)	1. Open and clear airway: modified jaw thrust.
Unequal chest rise	2. Expose chest.
Cyanosis (blue skin)	3. Take vitals.
Low BP	4. Lung sounds bilaterally.
Rapid, weak pulse (over 120)	5. Administer O_2.
Coughing blood	6. Rapid transport!
	7. Check vitals every 5 minutes.

Airway Obstruction

Signs and Symptoms	Management
Universal choking handsign	1. Heimlich maneuver.
Tension in neck and face muscles	
Panicky behavior	
Unconscious	

Asphyxia, Traumatic

Signs and Symptoms	Management
Distended veins head, neck, shoulder Shock Cyanotic (blue) tongue and lips Eyes bloodshot and bulging Coughing blood	1. Open and clear airway: modified jaw thrust. 2. Expose chest. 3. Administer high-flow O_2. 4. Assist breathing, as necessary. 5. Control bleeding. 6. Take vitals. 7. Rapid transport! 8. Take vitals every 5 minutes. 🕐

Asthma

Signs and Symptoms	Management
Noisy, labored breathing Wheezing Air hunger Anxiety Cyanosis (blue skin) Rapid pulse (over 120) Dry cough Sweating Exhaustion	1. Open and clear airway. 2. Rapid transport! In position of comfort. 3. Administer O_2 by Rx or as per local protocol. 4. Reassure.

Edema, Pulmonary

Signs and Symptoms	Management
Dyspnea (shortness of breath)	1. Open and clear airway.
Rising BP	2. Administer high-flow O_2.
Bulging neck veins	3. Assist breathing as necessary.
Noisy breath sounds	4. Rapid transport! Patient sitting.
Tachycardia (rapid pulse)	5. Reassure.
Anxiety	
Signs of shock	6. Take vitals
Distal edema (swelling of extremities)—late sign	every 5 minutes.

Emphysema, and Chronic Bronchitis (COPD)

Signs and Symptoms	Management
Noisy, labored breathing	1. Open and clear airway.
Wheezing	2. Loosen restrictive clothing.
Air hunger	3. Transport patient in sitting position.
Cyanosis (blue skin)	4. Administer O_2, 1–2 liters by nasal cannula or Rx (in case of trauma, administer high-flow O_2 by mask).
Bulging neck veins	
Coughing	
	5. Assist breathing, as necessary.

Emphysema, Subcutaneous

Signs and Symptoms	Management
Difficulty breathing	1. Open and clear airway.
Partial cyanosis (blue skin)	2. Expose chest.
	3. Transport.
Skin crackles on palpation	4. Administer high-flow O_2. No positive pressure!
	5. Assist breathing.
	6. Take vitals every 5 minutes. 🕐

Flail Chest

Signs and Symptoms	Management
Paradoxical respirations (uneven chest rise)	1. Open and clear airway: modified jaw thrust.
Guarding	2. Expose chest.
Crepitus (bone ends grating)	3. Take vitals.
	4. Administer high-flow O_2.
Swelling and discoloration at injury	5. Splint with pillows or patient's arm.
	6. Transport on injured side.
	7. Check vitals every 5 minutes. 🕐

Fractured Rib

Signs and Symptoms	Management
Guarding chest area	1. Open and clear airway: modified jaw thrust.
Shallow, cautious breathing	2. Expose chest.
Crepitus (bone ends grating)	3. Administer O_2.
Possible discoloration at injury	4. Sling and swath arm or use pillow to stabilize.
	5. Transport.
	6. Check vitals every 5 minutes. 🕐

Hemothorax

Signs and Symptoms	Management
Rapid, shallow breathing	1. Open and clear airway: modified jaw thrust.
Diminishing or absent breath sounds on one side	2. Expose chest.
Hemorrhagic shock	3. Administer high-flow O_2.
Coughing blood	4. Assist breathing.
	5. Treat for shock.
	6. Rapid transport!
	7. Take vitals every 5 minutes. 🕐

Pneumonia

Signs and Symptoms	Management
Hot, dry skin Elevated temperature Tachypnea (fast, noisy breathing) Heavy cough with phlegm and mucus Bubbly lung sounds, lower lobes	1. Transport in position of comfort. 2. Administer O_2. 3. Take vitals every 5 minutes. 🕐

Pneumothorax

Signs and Symptoms	Management
Dyspnea (shortness of breath) Diminishing or absent breath sounds on one side Uneven chest rise Sharp chest pain	1. Open and clear airway. 2. Expose chest. 3. Administer O_2. 4. Assist breathing as necessary. 5. Rapid transport! 6. Take vitals every 5 minutes. 🕐

Pneumothorax, Tension

Signs and Symptoms	Management
Tracheal deviation Dyspnea (shortness of breath) Intercostal retraction Distended neck veins Diminishing or absent breath sounds on one side	1. Open and clear airway: modified jaw thrust. 2. Expose chest. 3. Administer O_2. 4. Assist breathing, as necessary. 5. Treat for shock. 6. Rapid transport! 7. Take vitals every 5 minutes.

Ruptured Esophageal Varices

Signs and Symptoms	Management
Elevated pulse Pale or yellow color to skin Vomiting Hematemesis (vomiting of blood) No pain in abdomen Difficulty breathing	1. Open and clear airway.* 2. Administer O_2. 3. Suction, as necessary. 4. Treat for shock. 5. Rapid transport! 6. Take vitals every 5 minutes.

*Airway maintenance essential.

Separated Sternum

Signs and Symptoms	Management
Raid, shallow breathing Possible no breath sounds on one side Center of chest depresses on respiration Discoloration at site of injury	1. Open and clear airway: modified jaw thrust. 2. Expose chest. 3. Administer O_2. 4. Assist breathing, as necessary. 5. Stabilize with pillows. 6. Rapid transport! 7. Take vitals every 5 minutes.

Sucking Chest Wound

Signs and Symptoms	Management
Obvious open wound to chest Sucking and gurgling sounds	1. Open and clear airway: modified jaw thrust. 2. Expose chest. 3. Tape occlusive dressing over wound. 4. "Burp"; i.e., release one corner of dressing in case of tension pneumothorax. 5. Administer high-flow O_2. No positive pressure! 6. Rapid transport! In position of comfort. 7. Take vitals every 5 minutes.

4
Heart

Acute Myocardial Infarction (AMI)

Signs and Symptoms	Management
Generalized chest pain	1. Loosen clothing.
Pain radiates to arms and jaw	2. Open and clear airway.
Nausea and vomiting	3. Assess for breathlessness.
Diaphoresis (heavy sweating)	4. Check pulse.
	5. Apply CPR, as necessary.
	6. Administer high-flow O_2.
Dyspnea (shortness of breath)	7. Rapid transport! If patient conscious, semisitting position.
BP unreliable barometer	
Fear of dying	8. Maintain temperature.
Signs of shock	
Denial	9. Take vitals every 5 minutes. 🕐

Angina Pectoris

Signs and Symptoms	Management
Difficulty breathing	1. Administer O_2.
Substernal pressure	2. Transport.
Diaphoresis (heavy sweating)	
Short-term pain radiates to jaw or arms; 3–10 minute duration	3. Take vitals every 5 minutes. 🕐
Nausea	
Pain dissipates with rest	

Congestive Heart Failure

Signs and Symptoms	Management
Accelerated heart rate	1. Loosen clothing.
Noisy breathing	2. Open and clear airway.
Possible elevated BP	3. Assess for breathlessness.
Distended neck veins	4. Check pulse.
Dyspnea (shortness of breath)	5. Apply CPR, as necessary.
Fear of dying	6. Administer high-flow O_2.
Swelling of legs and/or feet	7. Rapid transport! If patient conscious, semisitting position.
Cyanosis (blue skin)	8. Maintain temperature.
Light red sputum or foam at mouth	9. Take vitals every 5 minutes. 🕐

Contusion, Myocardial*

Signs and Symptoms	Management
Chest pain	1. Open and clear airway.
Discoloration	2. Administer O_2.
Tachycardia (rapid pulse)	3. Assist breathing, as necessary.
Irregular pulse	4. Take vitals.
Distant or muffled heart sounds	5. Rapid transport!
Shock	6. Take vitals every 5 minutes. 🕐

*Caution: May lead to pericardial tamponade.

Contusion, Pulmonary

Signs and Symptoms	Management
Chest pain	1. Open and clear airway: modified jaw thrust.
Cyanosis (blue skin)	
Tachycardia (rapid pulse)	2. Take vitals.
Dyspnea (shortness of breath)	3. Administer high-flow O_2.
	4. Splint with pillow or patient's arm.
Imminent shock	5. Rapid transport! On injured side.
	6. Take vitals every 5 minutes. 🕐

Embolism, Pulmonary

Signs and Symptoms	Management
Difficulty breathing	1. Open and clear airway.
Stabbing chest pain	2. Administer high-flow O_2.
Tachycardia (rapid pulse)	3. Assist breathing, as necessary.
Coughing blood	4. Treat for shock.
Cyanosis (blue skin)	5. Rapid transport!
Decreasing BP	
Bulging neck veins	6. Take vitals every 5 minutes. 🕐
Signs of shock	

Pericardial Tamponade

Signs and Symptoms	Management
Distended neck veins	1. Open and clear airway.
Heart sounds distant and muffled	2. Administer O_2.
Pulse pressure equalizing	3. Assist breathing, as necessary.
Weak pulse	4. Take vitals.
Shock	5. Rapid transport!
	6. Take vitals every 5 minutes. 🕐

5
Abdomen

General Organ Injury

Signs and Symptoms	Management
Distended or rigid abdomen	1. Open and clear airway.
Progressive pain	2. Expose, search for wounds.
Patient generally in fetal position	3. Palpate four quadrants; check for pain, tenderness, rebound, hard or pulsing masses.
Guarding of abdomen	4. Take vitals.
Rapid, shallow breathing	5. Administer O_2.
Elevated pulse	6. Treat for shock.
Low BP	7. Rapid transport!
Nausea and vomiting	
Discoloration	8. Take vitals every 5 minutes. 🕐

Acute Abdominal Distress

Signs and Symptoms	Management
Abdominal distention	1. Open and clear airway.
Abdominal pain, local or diffuse	2. Take vitals.
Abdominal tenderness	3. Expose.
Rapid, shallow breathing	4. Palpate four quadrants; check for pain, tenderness, rebound, hard or pulsing masses.
Possible blood in vomit or stool	5. Administer O_2.
Elevated pulse	6. Treat for shock.
Referred pain	7. Rapid transport! In position of comfort.
	8. Take vitals every 5 minutes. 🕐

Bladder Injury

Signs and Symptoms	Management
Blood in urine Nausea and vomiting Pale skin Elevated temperature Inability to urinate or pain during urination	1. Open and clear airway. 2. Take vitals. 3. Expose. 4. Palpate four quadrants; check for pain, tenderness, rebound, hard or pulsing masses. 5. Administer O_2. 6. Treat for shock, if necessary. 7. Rapid transport! In position of comfort. 8. Take vitals every 5 minutes. 🕐

Kidney Injury

Signs and Symptoms	Management

Blood in urine
Pain, tenderness, and/or
   bruising on or around
   back
Shock
	1. Open and clear airway.
	2. Take vitals.
	3. Expose.
	4. Palpate four quadrants; check for pain, tenderness, rebound, hard or pulsing masses.
	5. Administer O_2.
	6. Treat for shock, if necessary.
	7. Rapid transport! In position of comfort.
	8. Take vitals every 5 minutes. 🕐

Peritonitis

Signs and Symptoms	Management
Elevated temperature Chills Pain radiating to shoulder from abdominal area No bowel sounds Abdominal pain	1. Open and clear airway. 2. Take vitals. 3. Expose. 4. Palpate four quadrants; check for pain, tenderness, rebound, hard or pulsing masses. 5. Administer O_2. 6. Treat for shock. 7. Rapid transport! In position of comfort. 8. Take vitals every 5 minutes. 🕐

Ruptured Hernia

Signs and Symptoms	Management
Abnormal lump in abdominal quadrants or groin Stabbing pain Nausea and vomiting	1. Expose. 2. Patient supine, knees drawn up. 3. Place support under knees. 4. Maintain temperature. 5. Transport. 6. Administer O_2. 7. Take vitals every 5 minutes. 🕐

6
Bones

Fractures

Signs and Symptoms	Management
EMT SLIPED	1. Expose.
Exposed bone ends	2. Check **CSM** (*c*irculation, *s*ensation, *m*otor function).
Muscle spasms	
Tenderness	3. Immobilize.
Shortening and swelling	4. Check **CSM** again.
Loss of motion and distal pulse	5. Transport.
Intense pain at site of injury	6. Take vitals every 5 minutes. ☾
Patient says it's broken	
Evident deformity	
Discoloration	

Internal Bleeding

Signs and Symptoms	Management
Discoloration	1. Open and clear airway.
Guarding on palpation	2. Administer O_2.
Swelling	3. Expose.
Pain at site of injury	4. Stabilize fractures, if any.
Blood from ears, nose, mouth, rectum, genitals	5. Treat for shock.
	6. Rapid transport!
Abdominal rebound, rigidity	7. Take vitals every 5 minutes. ☾
Abdominal muscle spasms	
Signs of shock	

Sprain (Bone-to-Bone)

Signs and Symptoms	Management
Torn ligaments	RIPE
No deformity	1. **R**est
Pain	2. **I**ce
Swelling	3. **P**ressure
Discoloration	4. **E**levation

Strain

Signs and Symptoms	Management
Torn muscle	1. Expose.
Searing pain at moment of injury	2. Check **CSM** (*c*irculation, *s*ensation, *m*otor function).
Some swelling	3. Immobilize (splint).
Some discoloration	4. Check **CSM** again.
	5. Transport.

7
Burns

Rule of Nines

Location	BSA Affected (%)	
	Adult	*Infant*
Head	9	18
Thorax		
Anterior	9	9
Posterior	9	9
Abdomen		
Anterior	9	9
Posterior	9	9
Arm (circumference)	9 (each)	9 (each)
Genitalia	1	1
Leg (circumference)	18 (each)	13.5 (each)

BSA = body surface area.

First Degree

Signs and Symptoms	Management
Epidermal layer burned and red Localized pain	1. Determine source of burning and remove. 2. Expose. 3. Cool burn with copious amounts of water. 4. Open and clear airway. 5. Administer O_2. 6. Take vitals. 7. Transport.

Second Degree

Signs and Symptoms	Management
Skin red; epidermal and dermal layers affected Injury swollen, wet Blisters Severe pain	1. Determine source of burning and remove. 2. Open and clear airway. 3. Expose. 4. Cool burn with copious amounts of water. 5. Assess percentage of burn using Rule of Nines (see p. 42). 6. Administer O_2. 7. Take vitals. 8. Cover burn with dry sterile dressing; separate fingers and toes. 9. Transport.

Third Degree

Signs and Symptoms	Management
Skin burned through Skin dry, brown, leathery, or white No pain Distinct odor	1. Determine source of burning and remove. 2. Open and clear airway. 3. Expose. 4. Cool burn with copious amounts of water. 5. Assess percentage of burn using Rule of Nines (see p. 42). 6. Administer O_2. 7. Take vitals. 8. Cover burn with dry sterile dressing; separate fingers and toes. 9. Transport.

Chemical Burn—Lime

Signs and Symptoms	Management
Variable degree of burn at given location Evidence of lime in area Told of patient contact with lime	1. Lightly brush lime off skin. 2. Flush with copious amounts of water. 3. Continue to flush until lime has been expelled.

Chemical Burn—*Not* Lime

Signs and Symptoms	Management
Variable degree of burn at given location Evidence of corrosives in area Told of patient contact with corrosives	1. Flush with copious amounts of water. 2. Continue to flush while exposing. 3. Continue to flush for 20 minutes.

Electrocution

Signs and Symptoms	Management
Decreased LOC (*level of* *c*onsciousness)	1. Safe scene. Be sure source of current has been shut off!
Irregular pulse	2. Maintain airway; C-spine precautions.
Abnormal or absent respirations	3. Rescue breathing or CPR, as necessary. (If patient unconscious, go to steps 7–9, then continue to steps 4–6 and 10.)
Cardiac arrest	
Burn injury at point of contact	
	4. Expose, and check for entrance and exit wounds.
	5. Apply dry sterile dressing to both areas.
	6. Check for possible fractures.
	7. Immobilize patient for possible spinal injury.
	8. Administer high-flow O_2.
	9. Rapid transport!
	10. Take vitals every 5 minutes. 🕐

Lightning

Signs and Symptoms	Management
Irregular pulse or cardiac arrest	1. Maintain airway; C-spine precautions.
Severe "scale" type burns at entrance and exit wounds	2. Rescue breathing and CPR, as necessary. (If unconscious, go to steps 6–8, then continue to steps 3–5 and 9.)
Loss of hearing, sight, and/or speech	3. Expose, and check for entrance and exit wounds.
Minimal bleeding from the ears	4. Apply dry sterile dressing to both areas.
Disorientation	5. Check for possible fractures.
Loss of consciousness	6. Immobilize patient for possible spinal injuries.
Abnormal respirations	7. Administer high-flow O_2.
Respiratory arrest	8. Rapid transport!
	9. Take vitals every 5 minutes. 🕐

Respiratory Burn

Signs and Symptoms	Management
Facial and nasal hair singed	1. Maintain airway.
Black residue in sputum	2. Patient in semireclined position.
Difficulty breathing, stridor, wheezing	3. Administer high-flow humidified O_2.
Cough	4. Take vitals.
Sooty, smoky smell to breath	5. Rapid transport!

8
Diabetes

Diabetic Coma
(Ketoacidosis or Hyperglycemia)

Signs and Symptoms

Rapid, weak pulse
Kussmaul respirations
    (deep, sighing,
    labored)
Acetone breath (sweet or
    fruity odor)
Patient appears drunk
Polydipsia (extreme
    thirst)
Polyuria (increased
    urinary output)
Warm skin
Nausea and vomiting
Signs and symptoms are
    gradual.

Management

1. Assess patient for stroke or
   cardiac signs and symptoms.
2. Look for Medic Alert tag.
3. Take history.

    DIED
    Diabetic?
    Insulin?
    Exercise?
    Diet?

4. If unsure of diabetic status,
   give glucose.
5. If patient unconscious, open
   and clear airway.
6. Administer high-flow O_2.
7. Airway management.
8. Treat for shock.
9. Rapid transport!

10. Take vitals
    every 5 minutes. ◷

Insulin Shock (Hypoglycemia)

Signs and Symptoms	Management

Signs and Symptoms

Elevated pulse
Normal breathing
No unusual breath odor
Possible seizure
Syncope (fainting)
Uncoordinated, weak
Patient appears drunk
Cool and clammy skin
No thirst or drooling
Diminished LOC (*level of c*onsciousness)
Rapid onset of signs and symptoms

Management

1. Assess patient for stroke or cardiac signs and symptoms.
2. Take history.

    DIED
    Diabetic?
    Insulin?
    Exercise?
    Diet?

3. Give glucose under tongue, if patient conscious.
4. If patient unconscious, clear and open airway.
5. Administer high-flow O_2.
6. Rapid transport!

7. Take vitals every 5 minutes. 🕐

9
Environmental Injuries

Air Embolism

Signs and Symptoms	**Management**
Blotchy or itchy skin	1. Open and clear airway; C-spine precautions.
Impaired vision	
General muscle and joint pain	2. Assess for breathlessness.
	3. Check pulse.
Diminished LOC (*level of c*onsciousness)	4. Apply CPR, as necessary.
	5. Administer O_2.
Light red sputum or foam at mouth	6. Position supine with head and chest lower than feet.
Nausea	7. Rapid transport!
Difficulty breathing	
Distal numbness and tingling	8. Take vitals every 5 minutes. 🕐
Personality change	

Decompression Sickness (Bends)

Signs and Symptoms	**Management**
Blotchy or itchy skin	1. Open and clear airway; C-spine precautions.
Severe headache	
Diminished LOC (*level of c*onsciousness)	2. Assess for breathlessness.
	3. Check pulse.
Impaired vision	4. Apply CPR, as necessary.
General muscle and joint pain	5. Administer O_2.
	6. Rapid transport!
Nausea	
Inability to urinate	7. Take vitals every 5 minutes. 🕐
Difficulty breathing	
Abdominal pain	
Serious central nervous system complaints	

Drowning—*No* Spinal Injury

Signs and Symptoms	Management

Respiratory arrest
Cardiac arrest
	1. Open and clear airway.
	2. Begin rescue breathing while moving patient to solid ground or board.
	3. Assess for pulselessness. Apply CPR, as necessary, regardless of elapsed time of immersion.
	4. Continue CPR until:
	  a. Patient revives.*
	  b. CPR taken over by equally or more experienced personnel.
	  c. Patient transported to hospital.
	  d. Totally exhausted, unable to continue.
	5. Maintain temperature.
	6. Rapid transport!

*If patient revives, administer high-flow O_2 and transport.

Drowning—*Suspected* Spinal Injury

Signs and Symptoms	Management

Respiratory arrest
Cardiac arrest
	1. Open and clear airway; C-spine precautions.
	2. Begin rescue breathing.
	3. Full spinal immobilization with long board.
	4. Assess for pulselessness. Apply CPR, as necessary, regardless of elapsed time of immersion.
	5. Continue CPR until:
	   a. Patient revives.*
	   b. CPR taken over by equally or more experienced personnel.
	   c. Patient transported to hospital.
	   d. Totally exhausted, unable to continue.
	6. Maintain temperature.
	7. Rapid transport!

*If patient revives, administer high-flow O_2 and transport.

Frostbite, Severe

Signs and Symptoms	Management
Skin white or blue/white	1. Move patient to warm place.
Stiff, frozen feel and appearance	2. Keep affected area frozen.*
Distal edema (swelling in extremities)	3. Rapid transport!
Loss of feeling in extremities	

After Treatment
  Blisters
  Skin turns purple
  Extreme pain

*If affected area has begun to thaw, rewarm in 110° F water during transport. Check local protocol.

Frostbite, Superficial

Signs and Symptoms	Management
Skin white, waxy	1. Move to warm place.
Epidermal layer stiff in extremities	2. Passive rewarming.
Distal edema (swelling in extremities)	3. Apply dry sterile dressing.
Possible blisters after treatment	4. Transport.
Loss of feeling in extremities	5. Take vitals every 5 minutes. ○

Heat Cramps

Signs and Symptoms	Management
Cramps in extremities or abdomen	1. Move to cool place.
Hot and sweaty	2. Elevate feet.
Nausea and vomiting	3. Liquids, sipped.
Dizziness	4. Administer O_2.
Elevated heart beat	5. Transport.
	6. Take vitals every 5 minutes. 🕐

Heat Exhaustion

Signs and Symptoms	Management
Nausea and vomiting	1. Move to cool place.
Dizziness	2. Take vitals.
Cool, clammy skin	3. Treat for shock.
Pallor	4. Administer O_2.
Decreasing BP	5. Liquids, sipped.
Headache	6. Cool patient artificially.
Pupils dilated	7. Keep patient from shivering. If patient begins shivering, reduce cooling process.
	8. Transport.

Heat Stroke

Signs and Symptoms	Management
Constricted pupils; later dilated	1. Move to cool place.
Hot, dry, red skin	2. Open and clear airway.
High body temperature (over 105° F)	3. Administer O_2.
Diminished LOC (*level of c*onsciousness)	4. Cool patient artificially.
Tachypnea (fast breathing); initially deep, becoming shallow, weak	5. Keep patient from shivering. If patient begins shivering, reduce cooling process.
Possible syncope (fainting)	6. Rapid transport!
Low BP	

Hypothermia

Signs and Symptoms	Management
Shivering (early sign)	1. Handle with extreme care!
Decreased **CSM** (*c*irculation, *s*ensation, *m*otor function)	2. Move to warm place.
	3. Remove wet clothing.
Diminished LOC (*level of c*onsciousness)	4. Insulate with dry clothing, blankets.
Deathlike appearance	5. Take vitals.
Decreasing vitals, pulse, respirations	6. Administer O_2.
	7. Passive warming.
Absence of shivering (late sign)	8. Sweet, warm liquids (no coffee, no liquor).
	9. Transport.

Note: The patient is not dead until warm and dead.

10
Bites, Drugs, and Poisons

Bites

Animal (Rabies)

Signs and Symptoms	Management
Punctured skin Discoloration Anxiety, panic	1. Airway management (facial bites). 2. Apply direct pressure to stop bleeding (dry sterile dressing). 3. Splint extremity. 4. Take vitals. 5. Reassure. 6. Transport. 7. Contact animal control with animal ID for rabies check.

Black Widow Spider

Signs and Symptoms	Management
Pinprick-type pain at first Muscle spasms, seizures Generalized pain Elevated temperature Nausea Rigid abdomen Headache Diaphoresis (sweating) Anxiety	1. Open and clear airway. 2. Rescue breathing or CPR, as necessary. 3. Clean wound. 4. Apply cold compresses. 5. Take vitals. 6. Administer O_2. 7. Transport. 8. Reassure. 9. Contact medical control with spider ID or description, if possible.

Brown Recluse Spider

Signs and Symptoms	Management
Progressive signs and symptoms over a period of hours to weeks "Bull's eye" discoloration at site of injury Flu-type symptoms Ulcer-type wound (late sign)	1. Open and clear airway. 2. Rescue breathing and CPR, as necessary. 3. Clean wound. 4. Apply cold compresses. 5. Take vitals. 6. Administer O_2. 7. Transport. 8. Reassure. 9. Contact medical control with spider ID or description, if possible.

Coral Snake (Venomous)

Signs and Symptoms	Management
Small scratches at injury site	1. Move patient from area of snake.
Minor or no pain	2. Lay patient down, keeping affected area lower than heart.
Little or no discoloration or swelling	
Symptoms come on slowly over period of hours	3. Maintain airway.
	4. Rescue breathing or CPR, as necessary.
Personality changes	5. Expose affected area, remove restrictive jewelry or clothing.
Drowsiness	
Impaired vision	6. Flush affected area with copious amounts of water.
Salivation	
Convulsions	7. Occlude superficial venous blood flow with constricting band lightly tied 4 in. from wound, toward heart (check local protocol).
Nausea	
	8. Splint affected extremity.
	9. Maintain temperature.
	10. Take vitals.
	11. Rapid transport!
	12. Contact medical control with snake ID or description, if possible.

Insect Sting

Signs and Symptoms	Management
Pinprick-type pain at first Redness Itchiness Swelling	1. Inspect for stinger at injury site. 2. Remove stinger with scraping motion using edge of card or knife. 3. Observe for signs of anaphylaxis (allergic reaction). 4. Rapid transport! 5. Treat for shock.

Pit Viper Snake (Venomous)

Signs and Symptoms	Management
Two obvious punctures side by side at site of injury	1. Move patient from area of snake.
Painful burning and swelling at injury	2. Lay patient down, keeping affected area lower than heart.
Ecchymosis (black and blue discoloration)	3. Maintain airway.
Inability of blood to clot	4. Rescue breathing or CPR, as necessary.
Numbness occurring over time	5. Expose affected area; remove restrictive jewelry or clothing.
Nausea	6. Flush affected area with copious amounts of water.
Diaphoresis (sweating)	7. Occlude superficial venous blood flow with constricting band lightly tied 4 in. from wound, toward heart (check local protocol).
Elevated pulse	8. Splint affected extremity.
Decreased BP	9. Maintain temperature.
Convulsions	10. Take vitals.
	11. Contact medical control with snake ID or description, if possible.

Drugs

General Overdose[a]

Signs and Symptoms

Altered LOC (*level of consciousness*)

Elevated or depressed pulse rate

High or low BP

Dilated or pinpoint pupils

Possible slurred speech

Possible seizures

Possible combativeness

Possible breath odor

Management

1. Safe scene.
2. Open and clear airway.
3. Rescue breathing or CPR, as necessary.
4. Take vitals.
5. Assess for other injury.
6. Contact medical control.

> SWATS
> **S**ubstance taken?
> **W**eight of patient?
> **A**ge of patient?
> **T**ime elapsed since taken?
> **S**yrup of Ipecac to induce vomiting?

7. Administer O_2 by nasal cannula.
8. Maintain temperature.
9. Rapid transport![b]
10. Reassure.

11. Take vitals every 5 minutes. 🕐

---

[a]Be aware that drugs or alcohol may not be the only problem, e.g., diabetic coma.

[b]Transport suspected substance and/or vomitus with patient.

Note: Do not induce vomiting without approval of medical control!

Alcohol

Signs and Symptoms	Management
Altered LOC (*level of consciousness*) Slurred speech Combative Breath odor Polyurea (increased urinary output) Evidence of substance	1. Safe scene. 2. Open and clear airway. 3. Rescue breathing; CPR, as necessary. 4. Take vitals. 5. Assess for other injuries. 6. Transport.

Hallucinogens (LSD, Mescaline, PCP)

Signs and Symptoms	Management
Altered LOC (*level of consciousness*) Hyperactivity Elevated pulse Dilated pupils Erratic behavior Hallucinations	1. Safe scene. 2. Open and clear airway. 3. Rescue breathing or CPR, as necessary. 4. Take vitals. 5. Assess for other injuries. 6. Contact medical control.

SWATS
Substance taken?
Weight of patient?
Age of patient?
Time elapsed since taken?
Syrup of Ipecac to induce vomiting?

7. Administer O_2 by nasal cannula.
8. Maintain temperature.
9. Rapid transport!*
10. Reassure.

11. Take vitals every 5 minutes. 🕐

---

*Transport suspected substance and/or vomitus with patient.
Note: Do not induce vomiting without approval of medical control!

Narcotics
(Codeine, Heroin, Methadone)

Signs and Symptoms	Management
Altered LOC (*level of consciousness*)	1. Safe scene.
Constricted pupils	2. Open and clear airway.
Depressed respirations	3. Rescue breathing or CPR, as necessary.
Cold and clammy skin	4. Take vitals.
Possible seizures	5. Stimulate patient.
No breath odor	6. Assess for other injury.
Drowsiness, lethargy	7. Contact medical control.
Evidence of substance in area	

SWATS

Substance taken?
Weight of patient?
Age of patient?
Time elapsed since taken?
Syrup of Ipecac to induce vomiting?

8. Administer O_2 by nasal cannula.
9. Maintain temperature.
10. Rapid transport!*

11. Take vitals every 5 minutes. ◯

---

*Transport suspected substance and/or vomitus with patient.
Note: Do not induce vomiting without approval of medical control!

Sedatives
(Sleeping Pills, Tranquilizers)

Signs and Symptoms

Altered LOC (*level of consciousness*)
Dilated pupils
Depressed respirations
Cold and clammy skin
No breath odor
Possible seizures
Drowsiness, lethargy
Evidence of substance in area

Management

1. Safe scene.
2. Open and clear airway.
3. Rescue breathing or CPR, as necessary.
4. Take vitals.
5. Assess for other injuries.
6. Contact medical control.

                SWATS
    Substance taken?
    Weight of patient?
    Age of patient?
    Time elapsed since taken?
    Syrup of Ipecac to induce vomiting?

7. Administer O_2 by nasal cannula.
8. Maintain temperature.
9. Rapid transport!*
10. Reassure.

11. Take vitals every 5 minutes. 🕐

---

*Transport suspected substance and/or vomitus with patient.
Note: Do not induce vomiting without approval of medical control!

Stimulants
(Amphetamines, Cocaine)

Signs and Symptoms	Management
Altered LOC (*level of consciousness*)	1. Safe scene.
Elevated body temperature	2. Open and clear airway.
Elevated BP	3. Rescue breathing or CPR, as necessary.
Dilated pupils	4. Take vitals.
Hyperactive	5. Assess for other injury.
Loss of appetite	6. Contact medical control.
Possible convulsions	
Possible hallucinations	
Possible combativeness	
Evidence of substance in area	

SWATS
Substance taken?
Weight of patient?
Age of patient?
Time elapsed since taken?
Syrup of Ipecac to induce vomiting?

7. Administer O_2 by nasal cannula.
8. Maintain temperature.
9. Rapid transport!*
10. Reassure.

11. Take vitals every 5 minutes. 🕐

---

*Transport suspected substance and/or vomitus with patient.
Note: Do not induce vomiting without approval of medical control!

Poisons

Poisoning by Ingestion

Signs and Symptoms	Management
Nausea and vomiting	1. Open and clear airway.
Abdominal pain	2. Contact medical control.
Diarrhea	
Polyuria (increased urinary output)	**SWATS**
	Substance taken?
Dilation or contraction of pupils	**W**eight of patient?
	Age of patient?
Drooling	**T**ime elapsed since taken?
Altered LOC (*level of consciousness*)	**S**yrup of Ipecac to induce vomiting?
Seizures	3. Rapid transport!*
Abnormal respirations	
Diaphoresis (heavy sweating)	4. Take vitals every 5 minutes. 🕐

*Transport suspected substance and/or vomitus with patient.
Note: Do not induce vomiting without approval of medical control!

Food

Signs and Symptoms	Management
Abdominal pain	1. Maintain airway.
Nausea	2. Transport.
Excessive bowel sounds	
Gas	
Diarrhea	
Fatigue	
History of last meal	

Pesticide

Signs and Symptoms

Salivation
Nausea
Abdominal pain
Dizziness
Headache
Chest discomfort
Lacrimation (tears)
Incontinence
General fatigue
Evidence of substance in
    area

Management

1. Handle patient with care. Do not contaminate yourself.
2. Maintain airway.
3. Administer high-flow O_2.
4. Expose patient.
5. Flush patient with copious amounts of water.
6. Contact medical control.

SWATS
Substance taken?
Weight of patient?
Age of patient?
Time elapsed since taken?
Syrup of Ipecac to induce vomiting?

7. Rapid transport!*

8. Take vitals
    every 5 minutes. ①

*Transport suspected substance and/or vomitus with patient.
Note: Do not induce vomiting without approval of medical control!

Petroleum

Signs and Symptoms	Management
Coughing or choking	1. Maintain airway.
Abnormal respirations	2. Take vitals.
Abdominal pain	3. Administer O_2.
Seizures	4. Contact medical control.
Irregular pulse	**SWATS**
Evidence of substance in area	**S**ubstance taken?
	Weight of patient?
Unusual breath odor	**A**ge of patient?
	Time elapsed since taken?
	Syrup of Ipecac to induce vomiting?
	5. Rapid transport!
	6. Take vitals every 5 minutes. 🕐

Note: Do not induce vomiting without approval of medical control!

Plant

Signs and Symptoms	Management
Pieces of plant evident on or around patient	1. Maintain airway.
Diarrhea	2. Take vitals.
Nausea	3. Administer O_2.
Salivation	4. Treat for shock.
Lacrimation (tears)	5. Contact medical control.
Burning in and around mouth	**SWATS**
	Substance taken?
Stomach ache	**W**eight of patient?
Abdominal pain	**A**ge of patient?
Hallucinations	**T**ime elapsed since taken?
Seizures	**S**yrup of Ipecac to induce vomiting?
Irregular pulse	6. Rapid transport!*
Elevated temperature	
	7. Take vitals every 5 minutes. 🕐

*Transport suspected substance and/or vomitus with patient.
Note: Do not induce vomiting without approval of medical control!

Poisoning by Inhalation

Signs and Symptoms

Nausea and vomiting
Diminished LOC (*level of c*onsciousness)
Noisy breathing
Dyspnea (shortness of breath)
Burns about face, singed facial hair
Discolored saliva
Chest pains
Watering eyes
Headaches
Cyanosis (blue skin)
Laryngeal edema (throat swelling)

Management

1. Patient supine with head elevated.
2. Loosen restrictive clothing.
3. Airway management and CPR, as necessary.
4. Administer high-flow O_2.
5. Rapid transport!
6. Contact medical control.

SWATS
   Substance taken?
   Weight of patient?
   Age of patient?
   Time elapsed since taken?
   Syrup of Ipecac to induce vomiting?

7. Check vitals every 5 minutes. 🕐

Note: Do not induce vomiting without approval of medical control!

Carbon Monoxide

Signs and Symptoms	Management
Pounding headache	1. Remove from source of fumes.
Nausea and vomiting	2. Airway management; CPR, as necessary.
Diminished LOC (*level of* consciousness)	3. Loosen restrictive clothing.
Blurred vision	4. Patient supine with head elevated.
Irritability	5. Administer high-flow humidified O_2.
Confusion	
Sleepiness	6. Rapid transport!
Seizures	7. Treat for shock.
Fainting and/or coma	
Cherry-red skin	8. Take vitals every 5 minutes. 🕐

11
Childbirth

Abortion, Spontaneous (Miscarriage)

Signs and Symptoms	Management
Vaginal bleeding or spotting Menstrual-like cramps	1. Take vitals. 2. Administer O_2. 3. Rapid transport!* 4. Reassure. 5. Take vitals every 5 minutes. 🕐

*Transport discharged material with patient.

Abruptio Placenta

Signs and Symptoms	Management
Rigid abdomen Minor bleeding Localized abdominal pain	1. Take vitals. 2. Administer high-flow O_2. 3. Shock position (patient supine with legs elevated). 4. Transport. 5. Take vitals every 5 minutes. 🕐

Breech Delivery, Buttocks

Signs and Symptoms	Management
Buttocks present before head.	1. Prepare for normal delivery. 2. Let progression of birth proceed naturally. 3. Support baby's body on hand while legs straddle arm. 4. If baby's head does not deliver within 3 minutes, open airway. 5. Rapid transport!

Breech Delivery, Limb

Signs and Symptoms	Management
Limb presents first.	1. Administer high-flow O_2. 2. Rapid transport!

Ectopic Pregnancy

Signs and Symptoms	Management
Severe abdominal pain Missed period Palpable mass in abdomen Decreased BP No difficulty breathing Vaginal spotting Elevated pulse Signs of shock	1. Take vitals. 2. Shock position (patient supine with legs elevated). 3. Maintain temperature. 4. Administer O_2. 5. Rapid transport! In position of comfort. 6. Take vitals every 5 minutes. 🕐

Placenta Previa

Signs and Symptoms	Management
Heavy bleeding from vagina Signs of shock No pain	1. Take vitals. 2. Shock position (patient supine with legs elevated). 3. Maintain temperature. 4. Administer O_2. 5. Rapid transport! In position of comfort. 6. Take vitals every 5 minutes. 🕐

Toxemia (Eclampsia)

Signs and Symptoms	Management
Progressing distal edema (swelling of extremities) Impaired vision Nausea Diminished LOC (*level of consciousness*) Headache Elevated BP (over 140/90) Pain in upper right quadrant Possible seizures Hyperflexive (exaggerated reflex)	1. Take vitals. 2. Alert medical control immediately. 3. Left lateral recumbent position. 4. Reassure. 5. Administer high-flow O_2. 6. Rapid transport! No lights, no sirens.

Umbilical Cord, Around Neck

Signs and Symptoms	**Management**
Umbilical cord presents around baby's neck.	1. Attempt to gently move cord over baby's head and/or shoulders. Do not pull cord! 2. If attempt fails and cord compromises baby's airway, position clamps 3 in. apart, and cut cord between clamps.

Umbilical Cord, Prolapsed

Signs and Symptoms	**Management**
Umbilical cord presents before baby.	1. Knee chest position (patient's buttocks raised above shoulders). 2. Administer high-flow O_2. 3. Gently wrap umbilical cord in sterile towel soaked in saline. 4. Rapid transport!

II

The Practical Exam

The practical portion of the EMT certification exam can take a whole day to complete, depending on the site and the number of trainees being tested. There are various stations that you must pass in the practical exam, and these are usually given in random order. However, within the context of each station, rigorous attention to sequence is essential. If you miss a step in a procedure or inadequately complete a sequence, you may fail that station and have to be retested. Within a station, moreover, if certain steps (highlighted here with black stars) are omitted or done improperly, the examiner will automatically fail you. That's why I wrote this book — to put the exact order of each station in a format for easy memorization and recall. In time, these procedures will become automatic to you. To help you remember them, key words have been capitalized, which, after study, will provide you with an instant memory check for the complete content of the step. A few commonly used acronyms (e.g., ABC for *A*irway, *B*reathing, *C*irculation) that will key your recognition of a particular step have also been included.

By no means should you be intimidated by the testing process. I've found that most examiners want you to pass. Even so, remember that some steps must be performed within certain time limits and that some require you to verbalize what you're doing. It's not enough to think to yourself, "Now I'm going to control any major bleeding I see." Examiners expect you to say *out loud*, "I am now observing for major bleeding. I will control any major bleeding that I see." In some stations, mannequins are used, in others, real people.

Station: CPR—First EMT

Step 1

While en route to the scene, **ASSEMBLE BAG VALVE MASK** with reservoir.

Step 2

CONNECT MASK to O_2.

Step 3

TURN ON O_2 to 15 LPM to deliver 100% O_2.

LPM = liters per minute.

Step 4 ⭐

CHECK EQUIPMENT
  POSITION face mask next to ear.
  LISTEN for O_2 flow.
  SQUEEZE BAG.
  FEEL for air flow.

Step 5

At scene, **ASSESS** patient responsiveness; **CONFIRM** unresponsiveness with second rescuer.

Step 6

OPEN AIRWAY. Head tilt, chin lift, **BUT** in case of spinal injury, modified jaw thrust instead.

Step 7

CHECK BREATHLESSNESS (3–5 seconds)
   LOOK for chest rise.
   LISTEN for breath sounds.
   FEEL for air flow on your cheek.

Step 8

INSERT AIRWAY of proper size.

(Verbalize for examiner, "Airway will not fit a mannequin.")

Step 9

APPLY FACE MASK securely.

Step 10

VENTILATE: Compress bag twice, watch for chest rise.

(Verbalize for examiner, "Mannequin's head must be hyperextended in order to ventilate.")

Step 11

CHECK PULSE (5–10 seconds) at carotid artery.

Step 12

If no pulse, **TELL PARTNER TO START CPR.**

(Correct ratio = 5 compressions per 1 ventilation)

Station (Continued): CPR— Second EMT

Step 13

KNEEL beside patient. **LANDMARK** on sternum— **POSITION** hands two fingers above costal arch.

(Shoulders should be directly above landmark, arms straight.)

Step 14

PACE
  80–100 compressions per minute
  5 compressions per cycle

DEPTH of compressions
  ½–1 in. for infants
  1–1½ in. for children
  1½–2 in. for adults

NO BOUNCING during compressions.
DO NOT REMOVE HANDS from patient's chest.

Step 15

COUNT OUT LOUD 5 compressions. **PAUSE** while partner ventilates. **FEEL** for chest rise. **RESUME** compressions and compression count.

(Helpful hint: As second EMT delivers compressions, first EMT checks carotid artery for stimulated pulse to ensure proper technique.)

Station:
O$_2$ Equipment

You will be tested on one of the three
O$_2$ devices that all EMTs must know
how to use:
    Nasal cannula
    Simple face mask
    Non-rebreather mask

Step 1

IDENTIFY EQUIPMENT called for by examiner.

Step 2

CONNECT EQUIPMENT to O_2.

Step 3

TURN ON O_2.

Step 4

ADJUST FLOWMETER
Nasal cannula
(prongs down)

COPD 1–2 LPM
4–6 LPM
24–44% O_2

Simple face mask

6–12 LPM
24–60% O_2

Non-rebreather mask
reservoir; allow reservoir
to fill before using

8–12 LPM
60–90% O_2

Step 5

PLACE EQUIPMENT NEXT TO YOUR EAR. Listen and feel for O_2 flow.

Step 6

APPLY EQUIPMENT to patient.

Station:
Traction Splint

CSM = Circulation
      Sensation
      Motor function

Step 1

EXPOSE the leg.
REMOVE shoe and sock.

Step 2

CHECK CSM (*c*irculation, *s*ensation, *m*otor function).

Step 3

INSTRUCT SECOND EMT to pull traction.

Minimize movement of leg.

Step 4

GAUGE SPLINT against uninjured leg; secure to proper length.

Step 5

SLIDE SPLINT under injured leg to base of buttocks.

Make sure foot stand is closed.

Step 6

APPLY ISCHIAL STRAP tightly and **PAD**, as necessary.

Step 7

RAISE FOOT STAND.

Step 8

SECURE ANKLE HITCH.

Step 9

USE TRACTION SPLINT to pull mechanical traction.

(Second EMT ceases manual traction.)

Step 10

IMMOBILIZE LEG with padded straps.

Step 11

CHECK CSM (circulation, *s*ensation, *m*otor function).

Station: Upper Extremity Splint

CSM = Circulation
      Sensation
      Motor function

Step 1

EXPOSE the injured arm.

Step 2

CHECK CSM (*c*irculation, *s*ensation, *m*otor function).

Step 3

CHOOSE APPROPRIATE EQUIPMENT (i.e., splints and/or cravats).

Step 4

APPLY AND SECURE splints on limb(s). Leave limb(s) in position found.

Step 5

IMMOBILIZE JOINTS above and below fracture.

Step 6

PAD KNOTS.

Step 7

MINIMIZE MOVEMENT of limb.

Step 8

CHECK CSM (circulation, sensation, motor function).

Station: Trauma, Primary Survey

ABC = *A*irway
      *B*reathing
      *C*irculation

Step 1

DETERMINE unresponsiveness.
CONFIRM with partner.

Step 2

A (*A*irway)
Modified jaw thrust; C-spine precautions.

Step 3

B (*B*reathing)
LOOK for chest rise.
LOOK for major chest injury.
LISTEN for breath sounds.
FEEL for air flow on cheek.

(3–5 seconds)

Step 4

C (Circulation)
Check for pulse at carotid artery (5–10 seconds).
Observe for major bleeding.
Treat bleeding, if found.

(Verbalize for examiner.)

Step 5

INSTRUCT PARTNER to maintain cervical stabilization.

(Verbalize for examiner.)

Step 6

SIZE AND FIT cervical collar.

(Verbalize for examiner.)

Step 7

CHECK level of consciousness
   AVPU = *A*lert
             *V*erbal stimuli
             *P*hysical stimuli
             *U*nresponsive

Step 8

SEARCH for life-threatening traumatic injury. Cut away clothing, as necessary.

Step 9

SEARCH for Medic Alert tags.

Step 10

TAKE VITAL SIGNS
   Pulse
   Respiration
   Blood pressure

(Verbalize taking vitals.)

Step 11

CHECK LUNGS bilaterally with stethoscope (six locations).

Step 12

ADMINISTER HIGH-FLOW O$_2$.

(Verbalize for examiner.)

Station: Trauma, Secondary Survey

Step 1

EXPOSE; cut away clothing.

(Verbalize for examiner.)

Step 2

HEAD AND NECK: Palpate for lumps, bumps, contusions, or bleeding.

Step 3

EARS AND NOSE: Check for fluids or blood.

Step 4

PUPILS
  PEARL = *P*upils
           *E*qual
           *A*nd
           *R*eactive to
           *L*ight

Step 5

MOUTH: Check for bleeding, vomitus, or foreign substances.

Step 6

CHECK: Clavicles
         Scapulae
         Ribs
         Sternum

Step 7

ABDOMEN: Check four quadrants for
  Pain
  Tenderness
  Rebound
  Guarding
  Hard masses
  Pulsing masses

Step 8

PELVIC REGION: Butterfly pelvic wings. Don't rock pelvis! Check groin.

Step 9

LEGS first, then **ARMS:** Check for fractures and swelling circumferentially.

CHECK CSM (*c*irculation, *s*ensation, *m*otor function).

Step 10

ASSISTED LOGROLL, C-spine precautions.

(Verbalize for examiner.)

Step 11

ENTIRE BACK, SPINAL COLUMN, AND BUTTOCKS:
Check for lumps, bumps, bleeding, or deformity.

Station: Military Anti-shock Trousers (MAST)

Step 1

VERBALIZE — RETAKE VITALS. For application of **MAST,** readings must be:
   Systolic blood pressure below 90
   Respirations above 20
   Heart rate above 110
   Lungs clear bilaterally

Step 2

REASONS TO QUESTION use of **MAST** (contraindications)
   Pulmonary edema
   Chest pain
   Hypothermic for 24 hours
   Abdominal evisceration
   Burns below level of **MAST**
   Late second trimester pregnancy
   Protruding foreign objects below level of **MAST**

Step 3

CHECK for sharp objects on or around patient.
REMOVE lower outer garments.

Step 4

ASSISTED LOGROLL, C-spine precautions.

Step 5

POSITION MAST under patient, three fingers below
  lowest rib.
OPEN valves.

Step 6

APPLY GARMENT in correct sequence:
  Right leg—80% velcro bond required
  Left leg—80% velcro bond required
  Abdomen—80% velcro bond required

Step 7

RECHECK top of **MAST** below lowest rib.

Step 8

CLOSE all valves.

Step 9

CONNECT foot pump.

Step 10

CONTACT Medical Control with latest vitals and patient profile prior to inflation.

Step 11

INFLATE MAST in correct sequence:
  Right leg
  Left leg
  Abdomen

(Make sure valves are open for chamber to be inflated and closed after inflation.)

Step 12

OPEN AND CLOSE each valve for correct inflation:
  50–100 mm Hg on gauge
  Relief valves pop
  Velcro crackles
  Over 100 systolic blood pressure

Step 13

RETAKE VITALS.

(Verbalize for examiner.)

Step 14 ★

DEFLATION CHECKPOINTS:
   Medical Control authorization required.
   Deflation rate minimum 20 minutes per chamber.
   Deflate abdomen first.

Station: Spinal Immobilization

Step 1

INSTRUCT PARTNER to maintain cervical stabiliza-tion.

Step 2

CHECK CSM (circulation, sensation, motor function) in extremities.

Step 3

SIZE AND FIT cervical collar.

Step 4

POSITION board.

Step 5

STRAP PATIENT at proper locations:

LONG BOARD
  ABOVE ankles
  ABOVE knees
  ACROSS pelvis
  BELOW armpit

SHORT BOARD
  ACROSS chest
  ACROSS waist

Step 6

PAD under buckles, as necessary.

Step 7

FILL VOIDS around legs and feet, head and neck, abdomen, and small of back with padding.

Step 8

SECURE HEAD.

Step 9

CHECK CSM (*c*irculation, *s*ensation, *m*otor function).

Appendix

Station: Semiautomated External Defibrillator (SAED)

Current U.S. Department of Transportation guidelines recommend that familiarization with SAED equipment and procedure be included in all EMT curricula. As a matter of course, this subject may be tested in some states. Check local protocol.

Step 1
Assess patient responsiveness. Patient unresponsive.

Step 2
Check breathlessness (5 seconds). No breathing.

Step 3
Insert airway.

Step 4
Ventilate: Compress bag twice, watch for chest rise.

Step 5
Check pulse at carotid artery (5–10 seconds).

Step 6
If no pulse, prepare for SAED application.

Step 7
Request advanced life support (ALS) response (check local protocol).

Step 8
Open pads and connect to SAED leads.

Step 9
Apply pads to clean dry skin. Shave chest, if necessary.

Step 10
Locate pads below the right clavicle, above nipple, and below the left breast so that pads create a direct line across the heart.

Step 11
Activate SAED to "Analyze" mode.

Step 12
SHOCK INDICATED.

Step 13
Shock at 200 joules.

Step 14
"Analyze" mode.

Step 15
SHOCK INDICATED.

Step 16
Shock at 200–300 joules.

Step 17
"Analyze" mode.

Step 18
SHOCK INDICATED.

Step 19
Shock at 360 joules.

Step 20
Check pulse at carotid artery (5–10 seconds).

Step 21
If no pulse, apply CPR for 1 minute.

Step 22
"Analyze" mode.

Step 23
SHOCK INDICATED.

Step 24
Shock at 360 joules.

Step 25
"Analyze" mode.

Step 26
SHOCK INDICATED.

Step 27
Shock at 360 joules.

Step 28
"Analyze" mode.

Step 29
SHOCK INDICATED.

Step 30
Shock at 360 joules.

Step 31
Check pulse at carotid artery (5–10 seconds).

Step 32
If no pulse, apply CPR for 1 minute.

Step 33
"Analyze" mode.

Step 34
SHOCK INDICATED.

Step 35
Shock at 360 joules three times.

Step 36
Continue sets of three shocks followed by CPR for 1 minute, after pulse check, until conversion ("NO SHOCK INDICATED") occurs.

Step 37
"NO SHOCK INDICATED"; apply CPR for 1 minute; reanalyze.

Step 38
"NO SHOCK INDICATED"; apply CPR for 1 minute; reanalyze.

Step 39
"NO SHOCK INDICATED"; apply CPR for 1 minute; reanalyze.

Step 40
Continue CPR, reanalyze every 1–2 minutes.

Step 41
Rapid transport!*

Step 42
CONTRAINDICATIONS
   Evidence of pulse
   Patient less than 12 years old or under 90 lbs
   Hypothermic patient

*Check local protocol.